Fatty Liver Disease

How to Prevent, Identify and Overcome NAFLD and NASH

Graham Pizzo

Disclaimer: *The information contained in this book is based on the research, opinions, and experiences of the author. It is not intended to replace professional medical advice or treatment. The reader should consult a physician regularly for any health issues and should always seek medical advice before modifying their diet, supplement, or exercise regimens. The author and publisher shall have no liability or responsibility to any person or entity for any loss or damage resulting from the information contained in this book. The information provided is general and may not apply to every individual. Any reliance on the information contained herein is solely at the reader's risk.*

Contents

Introduction-- **5**
Health Risks and Importance of Prevention and
Treatment-- 7
The Objectives of this Guide-----------------------------9

Chapter 1
The Basics of Fatty Liver Disease----------------------**11**
Definition and Difference between NAFLD
and NASH--- 11
Causes and Risk Factors of NAFLD--------------------13
Signs, Symptoms, and Diagnosis of NAFLD---------- 15

Chapter 2
Preventing Fatty Liver Disease---------------------- **18**
Making Dietary Changes----------------------------------18
Increasing Physical Activity and Exercise to
Prevent Fatty Liver Disease-----------------------------20
Maintaining a Healthy Weight and Losing
Weight if Needed to Prevent NAFLD------------------ 22
Managing Related Health Conditions to Prevent
the Progression of NAFLD------------------------------ 24

Chapter 3
Reversing Fatty Liver Disease Through Lifestyle-**27**
Different Dietary Approaches to Reverse Fatty
Liver Disease-- 27
Incorporating Intermittent Fasting to Help Reverse
NAFLD--- 29

The Importance of Quality Sleep and Stress
Management in Reversing Fatty Liver Disease-------- 31
How to Make Lifestyle Changes for Sustainable
Reversal of NAFLD--33

Chapter 4
Using Supplements to Improve Fatty Liver-------- 35
The Latest Research on Using Supplements to Help
Improve Fatty Liver Disease-----------------------------35
Safe Dosages and Potential Side Effects of Key
Supplements Used for Fatty Liver Disease------------- 37

Chapter 5
Medical and Surgical Treatments-------------------- 39
Medications for Treating Non-Alcoholic Fatty Liver
Disease---39
Bariatric Surgery and Other Surgical Procedures as
Potential Treatments Options------------------------------ 41
The Importance of Seeking Professional Medical
Advice on Fatty Liver Disease------------------------- 43

Chapter 6
Creating Your Fatty Liver Action Plan------------- 45
Assessing Specific Risks and Situations When
Creating a Fatty Liver Disease Action Plan------------ 45
Tips for Setting Diet, Lifestyle, and Supplement
Goals for Your Action Plan------------------------------ 47
Tips on Working with Your Doctor for Ongoing
Medical Care as Part of your Fatty Liver Disease
Management Plan--- 49
The Benefits of Joining a Fatty Liver Disease

Support Group--- 51

Conclusion--53
The Importance of Early Detection and Proactive
Lifestyle Changes--- 55
Motivation to Kickstart Your Action Plan Against Fatty
Liver Disease-- 56

Introduction

Non-alcoholic fatty liver disease (NAFLD) has reached epidemic proportions globally and is now one of the most common chronic liver diseases worldwide. Over the past few decades, NAFLD prevalence has risen in tandem with obesity rates. Currently, NAFLD affects an estimated 25% of people globally. In the United States, studies indicate up to 30% of adults and 10% of children have NAFLD.

Several factors have driven the NAFLD epidemic. The rising prevalence of obesity and type 2 diabetes are major risk factors, as NAFLD is closely associated with insulin resistance. Changes in dietary and lifestyle habits in much of the world have led to increased consumption of highly processed, high-calorie foods, as well as sedentary lifestyles and reduced physical activity. These factors contribute to weight gain and obesity, putting more individuals at risk for NAFLD.

Genetic susceptibility also plays a role. Certain ethnic groups, such as Hispanics, are at higher risk, independent of obesity and other risk factors. Prevalence also tends to increase with age, with the highest rates among those in middle age or older. The aging population in many countries may therefore contribute to more cases overall.

Beyond the sheer growth in cases, the severity of NAFLD has increased as well. As obesity rates have climbed, more patients are developing the inflammatory form of NAFLD known as non-alcoholic steatohepatitis (NASH). NASH can progress to permanent liver damage, including cirrhosis and liver cancer. This has led to NAFLD becoming a leading cause of liver transplants.

The societal and economic costs associated with the expanding NAFLD epidemic are substantial. NAFLD is now one of the top reasons for referrals to hepatology practices. It also contributes significantly to the burden of chronic liver disease and liver-related mortality. Addressing modifiable risk factors like obesity and insulin resistance at the population level will be key to reversing the tide of this epidemic. Lifestyle modifications, public health initiatives promoting healthy eating and exercise, and effective policies around food must be part of the solution.

Health Risks and Importance of Prevention and Treatment

NAFLD poses several health risks that make prevention and early treatment important goals. The first issue is the progression to more severe liver disease. Simple fatty liver disease can progress to NASH, which can then lead to permanent scarring of the liver (cirrhosis). Cirrhosis increases the risk of liver failure and liver cancer. These complications result in over 100,000 deaths per year attributed to NAFLD globally.

Beyond liver-related effects, NAFLD is linked to an increased incidence of type 2 diabetes, likely due to its association with insulin resistance. Multiple studies show those with NAFLD have a 2–5 times higher risk of developing diabetes compared to the general population. NAFLD also appears to increase cardiovascular disease risk by contributing to atherosclerosis, endothelial dysfunction, and cardiac abnormalities.

With obesity reaching epidemic proportions, the prevalence of NAFLD in children has also risen substantially. Obese children with NAFLD are at high risk of the disease progressing. Pediatric NAFLD is associated with premature atherosclerotic disease and other obesity-related complications.

Given these wide-ranging health consequences, screening those at high risk and intervening early with lifestyle changes or medication offers the best opportunity to alter the course of the disease. Even a 5–10% weight loss can improve steatosis, so weight management is first-line. Dietary changes to reduce processed carbohydrates and increase healthy fats may provide additional benefits. Exercise and activity are also important to promote metabolic health. Vitamin E and pioglitazone are pharmaceutical options with evidence for efficacy in NASH.

For advanced diseases, options are more limited but expanding. Liver transplantation is the only definitive treatment for end-stage liver disease. However, newer drugs like obeticholic acid show promise for fibrosis regression in NASH cirrhosis. Continued research into novel therapies is critical.

Halting further growth of the NAFLD epidemic will require broad public health and policy initiatives targeting obesity, nutrition, and lifestyle risk factors. Evidence-based recommendations around exercise, diet, and weight reduction should be widely disseminated. Consumer education will also be key. With awareness and preventative action, the tidal wave of NAFLD prevalence could be reversed.

The Objectives of this Guide

The goal of this book is to empower readers with up-to-date, evidence-based information and practical strategies regarding the prevention, management, and treatment of non-alcoholic fatty liver disease. As the global epidemic continues unchecked, education and awareness are urgently needed to help reverse the tide. This book aims to reach patients, loved ones, and anyone concerned about their liver health and equip them to take control.

Within these pages, readers will gain a solid understanding of the drivers of the NAFLD epidemic, its health implications, and current medical recommendations. The biology underlying the development of fatty liver will be explained in straightforward terms, outlining risk factors like obesity, poor diet, inactivity, and genetics. The latest data on prevalence across different ages, ethnicities, and geographical regions will underscore why NAFLD is a serious public health crisis warranting attention.

Most importantly, readers will learn the steps they can take to prevent or manage NAFLD. Practical lifestyle modification strategies will be detailed, including specific dietary approaches, tips for increasing physical activity, and evidence-based weight loss recommendations. The importance of losing just 5–10% of body weight will be emphasized as potentially reversing early-stage NAFLD. Safe exercise regimens and nutrient targets will be provided.

Available medical treatments for NAFLD will also be covered. Current pharmaceutical options, such as vitamin E, pioglitazone, and new experimental drugs, will be discussed. Guidance on screening tests and working with one's doctor will empower readers to take charge of monitoring their liver health.

This comprehensive resource aims to alleviate confusion and give readers confidence in what they can do to help combat this growing epidemic. From diet and exercise to the latest advances in treatment, the path to prevention and control of NAFLD will be laid out. This knowledge can inspire lasting lifestyle changes and better health. By equipping ourselves with information and making smart choices, we can start turning the tide against NAFLD.

Chapter 1

The Basics of Fatty Liver Disease

Definition and Difference between NAFLD and NASH

Non-alcoholic fatty liver disease (NAFLD) is defined as excessive fat accumulation in the liver of individuals who drink little to no alcohol. It encompasses a spectrum of conditions ranging from simple hepatic steatosis to non-alcoholic steatohepatitis (NASH), which can progress to cirrhosis and liver failure.

Hepatic steatosis is the buildup of fat in liver cells. It occurs when the rate of fat accumulation exceeds the rate of fat elimination. Typically, 5% or more of the liver by weight must be fat for a diagnosis of fatty liver. Steatosis alone is considered relatively benign.

NASH represents a more serious form of NAFLD characterized by liver inflammation and cell damage in addition to fat accumulation. The inflammation is triggered by a combination of factors including insulin resistance, oxidative stress, lipotoxicity from free fatty acids, dysregulation of the gut microbiota, and hormones that regulate appetite and metabolism.

While simple steatosis may never progress beyond excess fat, NASH can promote permanent scarring or fibrosis of the liver. Over time, this can advance to cirrhosis, which destroys the normal liver architecture and increases the risk of liver cancer. Therefore, while NAFLD refers broadly to fat in the liver, NASH denotes a progressive inflammatory condition posing greater health risks.

To differentiate between non-alcoholic fatty liver disease (NAFLD) with simple fat accumulation and non-alcoholic steatohepatitis (NASH), a liver biopsy is necessary. The biopsy shows inflammation and cell ballooning, which are the characteristic features of NASH. Although imaging tests and blood tests can be helpful, they cannot definitively diagnose NASH. However, high ferritin levels, elevated liver enzymes, the presence of diabetes or metabolic syndrome, and patterns on MRI or ultrasound suggesting fibrosis may give some clues for the diagnosis.

Not everyone with NAFLD develops NASH, and the factors that drive this progression are complex. Genetic differences, insulin resistance severity, diet, gut health, and other influences likely interplay. Many patients have simple steatosis that has remained stable for decades. But for some, NASH develops at varying speeds of advancement. Ongoing research aims to better predict prognosis and outcomes for individual patients.

NAFLD refers to any fat accumulation in the liver, apart from heavy alcohol use. NASH denotes progressive inflammation that can permanently damage the liver, leading to cirrhosis. It represents a more serious form of fatty liver disease, warranting close monitoring and proactive treatment when identified.

Causes and Risk Factors of NAFLD

The central driver of NAFLD is an excess of calories, particularly from processed carbohydrates and fats, along with inadequate physical activity, leading to overweight or obesity and fat accumulation throughout the body, including the liver. However, several other factors influence an individual's risk.

1. **Obesity:** Excess body fat, especially abdominal obesity, is closely linked to insulin resistance, which drives fat deposition in the liver. Over 70% of obese

adults have NAFLD. The more severe the obesity, the higher the risk. Even in children, obesity dramatically raises NAFLD risk.

2. **Type 2 Diabetes and Pre-diabetes:** Insulin resistance underlies both NAFLD and type 2 diabetes. Up to 70% of diabetics have NAFLD. Impaired fasting glucose and metabolic syndrome are also strong risk factors. Improving insulin sensitivity is key to managing NAFLD.

3. **Diet:** Diets high in processed carbohydrates like white bread, sugar, and sweetened beverages promote de novo lipogenesis, the direct production of fat in the liver. Likewise, diets high in saturated fats and trans fats contribute to NAFLD.

4. **Genetic Predisposition:** Variations in genes involved in lipid metabolism, insulin signaling, oxidative stress, and inflammation can increase NAFLD risk. Hispanics, Native Americans, and Caucasians have the highest prevalence.

5. **Gut Dysbiosis:** Small intestinal bacterial overgrowth and changes to gut microbiome composition are associated with NAFLD. Bacteria-produced endotoxins may drive liver inflammation.

6. **Medications:** Certain drugs like glucocorticoids, tamoxifen, amiodarone, methotrexate, and others can contribute to a fatty liver as a side effect.

7. **Smoking & Alcohol:** While light or moderate alcohol intake does not seem to increase risk substantially, heavy drinking can still contribute. Smoking is associated with more advanced fibrosis in NAFLD patients.

NAFLD arises from an interplay of behavioral, metabolic, genetic, and environmental factors. Obesity and insulin resistance are the primary drivers, but an individual's risks depend on the combination of these influences. Managing diet, activity, and weight remain the cornerstones for prevention.

Signs, Symptoms, and Diagnosis of NAFLD

In its early stages, NAFLD typically has no signs or symptoms. Most people are unaware that their liver fat is building up. As a "silent" disease, it often goes undiagnosed until it becomes more advanced.

As NAFLD progresses, some subtle symptoms may develop, including:

- Fatigue and malaise

- Upper right abdominal discomfort
- Enlarged liver detected on exam

However, these nonspecific symptoms could result from many other conditions. A definitive diagnosis requires testing. The main modalities for detecting and evaluating NAFLD are:

1. **Imaging:** Ultrasound, MRI, CT, or transient elastography can visualize fatty infiltration and identify patterns suggestive of advanced fibrosis. Ultrasound is most commonly used in the first line. No imaging modality can differentiate simple steatosis from NASH.

2. **Liver Enzymes:** Elevated ALT and AST point to liver injury but cannot determine the degree of damage. Levels may remain normal until the late stages for some patients.

3. **Fibrosis Markers:** Blood tests for biomarkers of fibrosis, like the FibroTest or ELF score, can estimate severity but cannot substitute for a biopsy.

4. **Liver Biopsy:** Remains the gold standard for confirming diagnosis and staging disease severity. A biopsy can distinguish NASH from simple

steatosis and determine the degree of inflammation and fibrosis.

Once NAFLD is identified, evaluation aims to determine whether NASH or cirrhosis is present, since more advanced disease warrants additional monitoring and treatment. Imaging and biopsy are the main methods. The presence of diabetes, high ferritin, or metabolic syndrome also raises suspicion for NASH.

Ongoing research seeks to develop better non-invasive diagnostics. MRI-based techniques show promise for quantifying liver fat percentages. Blood tests to detect biomarkers specific to NASH are in development but not ready for clinical practice.

For now, a combination of imaging, biopsy, and bloodwork is needed for accurate NAFLD diagnosis and staging. Since most patients lack symptoms until late stages, screening those at high risk is important to catch progression early when lifestyle interventions can help prevent cirrhosis.

Chapter 2

Preventing Fatty Liver Disease

Making Dietary Changes

Diet plays a central role in both the development and prevention of NAFLD. Limiting processed carbohydrates, added sugars, and unhealthy fats can help reverse fat accumulation in the liver. Key dietary changes include:

1. **Reduce added sugars:** Foods and drinks high in added sugars like soda, candy, baked goods, and condiments promote de novo lipogenesis and should be minimized. The WHO recommends limiting added sugars to under 5% of total calories.

2. **Choose whole grains:** Refined grains act similarly to added sugars in the liver. Opt for whole grains like brown rice, quinoa, oats, and 100% whole wheat bread instead of processed grains.

3. **Increase fiber:** Soluble fiber from fruits, vegetables, beans, nuts, and oats helps improve

blood sugar control and may benefit the gut microbiota. Strive for 25–30 grams of fiber daily.

4. **Limit processed carbohydrates:** Pastries, chips, white bread, and other high-glycemic processed carbs contribute to NAFLD. Reduce portion sizes and frequency.

5. **Pick healthy fats:** Swap saturated and trans fats for monounsaturated fats like olive oil, avocado, and nuts, which may protect the liver. Include omega-3-rich foods like fatty fish.

6. **Eat more produce:** Fruits and vegetables are low in calories and rich in antioxidants, vitamins, minerals, and fiber. They provide nutrients that benefit liver health.

7. **Drink water:** Stay well hydrated by limiting sweetened beverages. For those with diabetes, manage their carbohydrate intake.

8. **Use herbs or spices:** Turmeric, ginger, garlic, and cinnamon have anti-inflammatory effects and can reduce the need for added salt or sugar.

9. **Portion control:** Even healthy foods should be eaten in moderation if you are trying to lose weight. Limit portions, especially of calorie-dense foods.

10. **Cook at home:** Preparing meals at home enables better control over ingredients and portions compared to eating out.

Making these evidence-based diet changes consistently can promote weight loss and improve metabolic health, helping reverse NAFLD. Work with a nutritionist or doctor if you need additional guidance tailoring dietary changes to your health status and preferences.

Increasing Physical Activity and Exercise to Prevent Fatty Liver Disease

Along with dietary changes, increased physical activity and exercise are critical components for preventing and managing NAFLD. Exercise confers several benefits:

- Burns calories to facilitate weight loss and maintenance. A negative energy balance is key to reducing excess fat, including in the liver. Even a 5–10% weight reduction can significantly improve NAFLD.
- Builds muscle mass, which has a metabolic benefit; more muscle increases resting energy expenditure. Loss of muscle during dieting can slow the

metabolism. Resistance training helps retain muscle.

- Improves insulin sensitivity and lowers blood sugar, countering risk factors for NAFLD progression to NASH and cirrhosis. Exercise enhances insulin signaling and glucose uptake in muscle tissue.
- Reduces chronic inflammation that can lead to liver damage in NAFLD. Physical activity has systemic anti-inflammatory effects.
- Can help reduce liver fat independently of weight loss. Some research shows exercise alone decreases intrahepatic fat content.

The CDC recommends 150 minutes per week of moderate-intensity physical activity such as brisk walking. Adding muscle-strengthening exercise at least two days per week provides further benefits. Those with obesity may need to exceed 200–300 minutes per week for substantial weight loss.

Start slowly and build up duration and intensity gradually. Walking is an easy activity to begin with. Swimming, cycling, hiking, dancing, sports, and yardwork are other options. Strength training with body weights, bands, or weights helps retain muscle. Consider high-intensity interval training once a baseline of endurance is built.

Staying motivated long-term is challenging. Having a partner to exercise with provides social support. Varying workouts prevent boredom. Setbacks are normal; just get back on track. Monitor your progress by tracking calories, weight, or other metrics. Most importantly, find activities you enjoy and turn exercise into a habit. Increased physical activity paired with diet improvements can make a real difference in NAFLD prevention and treatment.

Maintaining a Healthy Weight and Losing Weight if Needed to Prevent NAFLD

Achieving and maintaining a healthy body weight is one of the most effective ways to prevent and manage NAFLD. Since obesity is closely linked to insulin resistance and metabolic dysfunction driving fatty livers, weight loss should be a priority for overweight people.

Modest weight reduction of just 5–10% of body weight has been shown to significantly decrease liver fat content and reverse some of the liver damage in NAFLD. Greater weight loss provides further improvement. Avoiding weight gain is also crucial for sustained benefits.

Aim for a slow, steady rate of weight loss through sustainable lifestyle modifications. Very low-calorie diets or extreme regimens rarely lead to long-term success. A loss of 0.5 to 2 pounds per week is reasonable for most. Calories should come from whole, minimally processed foods, emphasizing produce, lean proteins, fiber, and healthy fats. Portion control is key.

Increasing physical activity is essential for weight loss and maintenance. Aerobic exercise for 150–300 minutes per week plus strength training provides the calorie deficit and metabolic boost to facilitate fat loss. Find activities you enjoy and that fit your current fitness level. Social support can bolster motivation.

Outside support through weight loss programs or counseling can help. Food logs, apps, and wearable devices that track activity and calories can promote awareness and keep you on track. Check-ins with your doctor to monitor progress are wise. Consider anti-obesity medications or bariatric surgery if other measures are unsuccessful.

Above all, make changes slowly and be consistent. It often takes many months to reach weight-loss goals. Don't get discouraged by plateaus. Focus on building healthy habits that allow weight maintenance once your target is met.

Remember, you don't have to become underweight. Reaching a body mass index within the normal range (18.5 to 24.9) significantly reduces health risks. Even losing just 10% of excess body fat can have measurable benefits. Improving your diet, increasing activity, and achieving a healthy weight provide the best defense against NAFLD progression.

Managing Related Health Conditions to Prevent the Progression of NAFLD

Since NAFLD is closely tied to obesity, insulin resistance, and other aspects of metabolic syndrome, properly managing related conditions is important for prevention and treatment. Key strategies include:

1. **Control blood sugar levels:** Monitoring blood glucose through HbA1c tests and adhering to treatment plans for type 2 diabetes or prediabetes can reduce insulin resistance and lower the risk of NAFLD progression.

2. **Optimize cholesterol:** Statin therapy may be appropriate for some patients to manage LDL and triglyceride levels. Fish oil supplements can help raise HDL.

3. **Lower blood pressure:** Hypertension is associated with more advanced NAFLD. Lifestyle changes and medications to achieve target blood pressure can reduce cardiovascular risks.

4. **Treat sleep apnea:** Obstructive sleep apnea exacerbates insulin resistance and systemic inflammation, which impact NAFLD severity. Use of CPAP and weight loss help.

5. **Consider medications:** Metformin and pioglitazone have shown efficacy in improving NAFLD, particularly for diabetes patients. Discuss options with your doctor.

6. **Don't smoke:** Smoking worsens cardiovascular risks and may accelerate NAFLD progression. Quitting improves outcomes.

7. **Moderate alcohol consumption:** While heavy drinking clearly worsens any liver condition, modest consumption has not been shown to impact NAFLD and may even provide some benefit, according to recent studies. Discuss safe levels with your provider.

8. **Stay on top of routine health screening:** Follow guidelines for colon cancer screening, bone density

tests, breast and prostate exams, etc. to enable early detection of other conditions.

9. **Reduce stress:** While not fully proven, high stress may exacerbate NAFLD through its effects on metabolism and inflammation. Healthy coping skills are wise.

Making positive changes to related health factors enhances overall well-being and can slow NAFLD progression. Work closely with your healthcare team to develop a comprehensive management plan.

Chapter 3

Reversing Fatty Liver Disease Through Lifestyle

Different Dietary Approaches to Reverse Fatty Liver Disease

Several evidence-based dietary strategies can facilitate fat loss in the liver and help reverse NAFLD. Common approaches include:

1. **Low-Carb Diets:** Limiting carbohydrate intake to under 30–50 g daily stimulates fat burning. Very low-carb ketogenic diets may rapidly reduce liver fat, but sustainability is an issue for many. Moderately low-carb diets are likely preferable long-term.

2. **Mediterranean Diet:** Emphasizes plant foods, healthy fats like olive oil and nuts, fish, and moderate dairy, and limits red meat and processed foods. Shown to reduce liver fat, inflammation, and fibrosis markers in NAFLD patients.

3. **Intermittent Fasting:** Alternating intervals of fasting and eating may help reverse NAFLD, even without major calorie reduction. Time-restricted feeding to limit intake to 8 hours per day is one popular approach.

4. **DASH Diet:** Dietary Approaches to Stop Hypertension focuses on fruits, vegetables, lean protein, low-fat dairy, whole grains, nuts, and limits sodium and sweets. Can aid weight loss and improve liver tests.

5. **Low-Glycemic Diet:** Choosing foods that minimize spikes in blood sugar can enhance satiety and reduce insulin resistance. Include protein, healthy fats, and fiber at meals.

6. **Plant-Based/Vegetarian:** Emphasizing produce, nuts, seeds, beans, and whole grains and limiting processed food, saturated fat, and refined carbs promotes weight loss and metabolic health.

The key is finding a style of healthy eating you can maintain long-term that promotes weight management or loss if needed. Work with a nutritionist or doctor to find the eating pattern that best fits your preferences and health goals. Monitor triglycerides, liver enzymes, glucose, and inflammation markers to gauge impact. Small tweaks over time can produce big changes in reversing NAFLD.

Incorporating Intermittent Fasting to Help Reverse NAFLD

Intermittent fasting involves alternating periods of fasting with eating windows. This pattern of intermittent calorie restriction may provide benefits for reversing NAFLD beyond standard continuous calorie reduction.

There are several popular fasting protocols. The 16:8 method entails fasting for 16 hours per day and restricting food intake to an 8-hour window, typically between noon and 8 p.m.Alternate-day fasting calls for 500 calories on the fasting day, alternating with an unrestricted day. The 5:2 method involves two days per week of restricted calories (500–600 calories) and five days of eating without counting calories.

Research on obese adults with NAFLD shows intermittent fasting can significantly reduce intrahepatic fat content and improve the NAFLD Activity Score on biopsy after just 8–12 weeks. Improvements exceed those typically seen with a standard daily calorie reduction alone. Fasting triggers fat burning for fuel and may modulate liver fat metabolism.

Intermittent fasting may work by:

- Lowering insulin levels leads to the lipolysis of fat stores.
- Activating autophagy and cellular repair processes
- Beneficially altering the gut microbiome

Adherence can be challenging with strict alternate days or 5:2 fasting. The 16:8 method with a consistent 8-hour eating window each day may be a more sustainable long-term option. Work up slowly from 12 hours to eventually 16 hours of fasting daily. Continue to emphasize healthy food choices in the eating window.

Those with diabetes or on medications should discuss fasting regimens with their doctor and monitor blood sugar closely to ensure safety. Start conservatively and adjust accordingly. Intermittent fasting, along with daily activity, a healthy diet, and weight management, offers a promising way to reverse NAFLD.

The Importance of Quality Sleep and Stress Management in Reversing Fatty Liver Disease

Alongside diet and exercise, improving sleep quality and managing stress levels are often overlooked but important components of an overall lifestyle approach to reverse NAFLD.

Poor sleep is linked to obesity, impaired glucose metabolism, and higher risks of chronic diseases, including NAFLD. Getting sufficient deep, restorative sleep enables proper metabolic functioning and cellular repair processes. Aim for 7-9 hours a night for adults and 8-10 hours for children and teenagers.

Practice good sleep habits like keeping a consistent bedtime and wake time, limiting blue light exposure in the evenings, and making sure your bedroom is cool, dark, and quiet. Reduce consumption of stimulants like caffeine and nicotine close to bedtime. Treat any underlying sleep disorders, like sleep apnea.

Relaxation techniques before bed, like taking a warm bath, reading, gentle yoga, or meditation, can help wind down. Cognitive behavioral therapy for insomnia provides tools to

5. **Involve others:** Share your goals and progress with family and friends, or post on social media. Social support improves adherence and accountability.

6. **Address obstacles:** Identify your unique barriers to change, like the environment, time, costs, or skills. Seek solutions rather than excuses. Enlist professional support if needed.

7. **Focus on how you feel:** Connect these changes to improved energy, sleep, mood, or lab markers. Feelings reinforce behavior better than distant health threats.

8. **Allow flexibility:** Allow for periodic indulgences and "imperfect" days. Rigid perfectionism leads to failure. Get back on track for the next meal or day without self-judgment.

9. **Shift your mindset:** Consider yourself someone who lives healthfully rather than forcing temporary changes. Let healthy choices define your identity.

Make healthy living a rewarding part of your daily life and be patient with yourself while keeping long-term health goals in mind.

Chapter 4

Using Supplements to Improve Fatty Liver

The Latest Research on Using Supplements to Help Improve Fatty Liver Disease

Some nutritional supplements have been investigated for potential benefits for NAFLD, but research is still emerging. Some of the most promising include:

1. **Vitamin E:** Large randomized trials found high-dose vitamin E (800 IU/day) improved liver histology and resolved NASH in a significant portion of non-diabetic adults. However, long-term safety is debated.

2. **Omega-3 Fatty Acids:** Fish oil supplements appear to decrease liver fat, improve insulin sensitivity, and lower triglycerides. DHA may be the key component. Benefits are maximized at doses over 2 grams per day.

3. **Milk Thistle:** Silymarin, the active compound in milk thistle, has antioxidant and anti-inflammatory properties. Meta-analyses show it improves liver enzymes and steatosis, but better studies are needed.

4. **CoQ10:** This antioxidant and electron transporter may improve NAFLD by enhancing mitochondrial function. Doses around 100–200 mg per day normalized liver enzymes in small studies. Larger trials are underway.

5. **Curcumin:** The polyphenol in turmeric has anti-inflammatory, antioxidant, and anti-fibrotic effects. Curcumin showed improvements in liver fat, fibrosis, and enzymes in several randomized studies.

6. **Probiotics:** Certain probiotic strains appear to improve gut health and permeability, lower inflammatory markers, and decrease liver fat. But optimal mixtures and doses remain unclear.

Remember, supplements should complement, not replace, lifestyle interventions like diet and exercise. Work closely with a doctor before starting supplements. Effects likely depend on the individual and stage of fatty liver disease. More rigorous research is needed to clarify the roles of various supplements in NAFLD treatment.

Safe Dosages and Potential Side Effects of Key Supplements Used for Fatty Liver Disease

When using supplements, it's important to understand appropriate dosing as well as potential side effects and drug interactions.

1. **Vitamin E:** Doses used in major clinical trials showing benefits for NASH were 800 IU per day. However, the NIH recommends an upper limit of 1,000 IU daily over the long term due to the increased risk of bleeding and hemorrhagic stroke. High-dose vitamin E may also increase prostate cancer risk in men.

2. **Milk Thistle:** Silymarin doses in studies range widely from 200 to 700mg daily. Milk thistle is generally well tolerated, with occasional side effects like gastrointestinal upset and headaches. Very high doses may cause laxative effects. People with ragweed allergies can be allergic to milk thistle.

3. **Turmeric:** Most clinical trials use curcumin doses of around 1000mg per day. Curcumin absorption can be enhanced by formulations like phytosomes. Up to 8 grams per day appears safe in studies, but high doses may increase bleeding risk. Can cause

GI side effects like reflux, nausea, or diarrhea, especially when taken on an empty stomach.

4. **Omega-3 Fatty Acids:** Doses of 2-4 grams daily of combined EPA and DHA appear most effective for NAFLD and triglyceride lowering. Can cause a fishy aftertaste and gastrointestinal side effects. Those on blood thinners should exercise caution.

5. **CoQ10:** Doses up to 500mg daily appear well tolerated, but little safety data exists long-term or at high doses. Headaches, nausea, and gastrointestinal discomfort are occasional side effects. Could interact with cholesterol or blood pressure medications.

Remember, none of these supplements have been approved specifically for NAFLD treatment. Work closely with your doctor to discuss the latest evidence, establish a need, and determine a safe dosage tailored to your health status. Lifestyle therapies remain foundational.

Chapter 5

Medical and Surgical Treatments

Medications for Treating Non-Alcoholic Fatty Liver Disease

While lifestyle modification is first-line, several medications may be appropriate as additional therapy for certain NAFLD patients:

1. **Metformin:** This diabetes drug improves insulin sensitivity and may reduce liver fat content. It is often used off-label in non-diabetic patients with NASH, but its long-term efficacy is debated.

2. **Pioglitazone:** This insulin-sensitizing agent helps resolve NASH and improve fibrosis markers in many patients, with good longer-term data. However, it can cause weight gain.

3. **GLP-1 agonists:** Liraglutide and other injectable GLP-1 analogs benefit glucose control and may

reduce liver fat, inflammation, and fibrosis progression in NASH.

4. **Statins:** While used primarily for high cholesterol, statins appear to benefit NAFLD. Atorvastatin and rosuvastatin improved liver histology in small trials. Larger studies are underway.

5. **Vitamin E:** As an antioxidant, high-dose vitamin E (800 IU/day) has been shown to resolve NASH in nondiabetic adults. Long-term safety concerns exist, however.

6. **Ursodeoxycholic acid (UDCA):** Several trials found improvement in liver enzymes with UDCA but no histologic benefit. Routine use is not currently recommended.

7. **Newer agents:** Obeticholic acid improved fibrosis in NASH cirrhosis trials. Elafibranor, selonsertib, and other investigative drugs have shown promising results for NASH in phase 2 and 3 trials so far.

No pharmacotherapy is yet approved specifically for NAFLD or NASH. Medications may be appropriate for certain patients with aggressive diseases, especially those with diabetes or metabolic syndrome. Pioglitazone and GLP-1 agonists have the strongest evidence currently.

Continued research into novel agents offers hope for expanding treatment options.

The benefits and risks of any medication should be carefully considered. Work closely with a hepatologist or gastroenterologist to determine if pharmaceutical therapy is warranted alongside continued lifestyle management.

Bariatric Surgery and Other Surgical Procedures as Potential Treatments Options

For patients with severe obesity who are not amenable to lifestyle changes or medications, bariatric or metabolic surgery may be an option to treat NAFLD. Procedures like gastric bypass, sleeve gastrectomy, and gastric banding produce significant weight loss, which is key for reducing liver fat.

Multiple studies show major improvement and even resolution of fatty liver disease after bariatric surgery. Over 90% of patients show decreases in steatosis, with higher rates of NASH resolution compared to lifestyle or medications alone. Improvements likely result from surgery-induced caloric restriction, altered gut hormones favoring weight loss, and metabolic changes independent of weight loss.

However, bariatric surgery is not without risks, including infection, blood clots, and nutritional deficiencies requiring close monitoring. Strict criteria also determine eligibility based on BMI and comorbidities. For appropriate candidates, bariatric surgery offers perhaps the most rapid and effective means of reversing NAFLD.

For end-stage NASH cirrhosis patients awaiting transplant, newer procedures like aspiration microbial devitalization may help. This outpatient technique uses liposuction to remove some fat tissue, followed by the instillation of a detergent solution into the liver, which triggers regeneration. Small trials show significant histologic improvement in fibrosis after 6 months.

Partial hepatectomy is also being explored, where 30–70% of the cirrhotic liver is surgically resected, prompting the regrowth of non-cirrhotic tissue. Pilot data is promising, but larger controlled trials are needed.

While not yet widely used, surgical approaches beyond bariatric procedures are an intriguing area of study for advanced NASH cirrhosis. Such techniques may help delay or even avoid liver transplants. Patients should participate in research protocols and not undergo unproven procedures prematurely. Discuss all surgical options thoroughly with your hepatology team.

The Importance of Seeking Professional Medical Advice on Fatty Liver Disease

If you've been diagnosed with NAFLD or suspect you may be at risk, seeking guidance from a qualified medical professional is highly recommended. NAFLD ranges from mild to severe, with the potential for progression. Having an expert oversee your care provides the best chance of successful management.

Start with your primary care physician for an initial evaluation. They can check bloodwork to look for indicators of advanced liver disease and perform imaging such as an abdominal ultrasound to detect fatty infiltration. Based on the results, your PCP may advise dietary changes and increased physical activity.

For moderate-to-severe cases, a referral to a gastroenterologist or hepatologist who specializes in liver disease is wise. These specialists can provide a more extensive assessment through tests like transient elastography, liver biopsy, and advanced imaging to accurately grade the level of damage. They also offer guidance on when advanced medications or interventions may be appropriate.

Dietitians or nutritionists can also help create an individualized eating plan that addresses the dietary drivers of your liver disease while ensuring balanced nutrition. Exercise physiologists can tailor activity recommendations to your needs and limitations. Mental health counselors assist with stress reduction techniques.

Support groups, either in-person or online, provide community and allow you to learn from others navigating fatty liver disease. Leading centers also participate in clinical trials of emerging therapies you may be eligible for.

Stay engaged and informed about your care. Learn as much as you can about NAFLD so you can best communicate with your treatment team. Together, develop a comprehensive management plan you feel ready to implement. Monitoring and adapting the plan periodically helps sustain progress. With professional guidance, you can gain control over NAFLD and achieve the healthiest outcome possible.

Chapter 6

Creating Your Fatty Liver Action Plan

Assessing Specific Risks and Situations When Creating a Fatty Liver Disease Action Plan

The first step in creating your fatty liver disease action plan is taking an honest assessment of your particular risks and current situation. Factors to consider include:

1. **Weight and Body Composition:** What is your current weight, BMI, and body fat percentage? Being overweight or obese significantly increases the risk of NAFLD as well as the potential for progression to NASH. Even mild to moderate excess weight contributes to a fatty liver.

2. **Diet Quality:** What does your typical diet look like? Diets high in processed carbs, added sugars, saturated fats, and fiber promote NAFLD. Review your eating patterns for nutritional deficiencies or excesses.

3. **Physical Activity Levels:** How much exercise and movement do you get each day and week? Sedentary lifestyles and inactivity raise risks for insulin resistance and NAFLD. Aim for 150–300 minutes per week of moderate activity.

4. **Related Health Conditions:** Do you have obesity, prediabetes, type 2 diabetes, metabolic syndrome, hypertension, or sleep apnea? These interrelated conditions often coexist with NAFLD and heighten risks.

5. **Lab Results:** What are your recent lab tests showing? Elevated liver enzymes, triglycerides, fasting glucose, HbA1c, and low HDL point to metabolic dysfunction. Trends matter more than single tests.

6. **Imaging/Biopsy Results:** Ultrasound, MRI, or biopsy gives direct insight into the degree of fat infiltration, inflammation, and fibrosis. These help with stage severity and prognosis.

7. **Genetic Factors:** A family history of NAFLD may indicate a genetic predisposition. Ethnic background plays a role, with Hispanics and Caucasians at higher risk.

Honestly confronting your risks and starting point allows you to make informed decisions and practical goals for reversing course. Track relevant metrics over time to gauge progress. Courses are correct when needed. Enlist your care team's help in analyzing your health status.

Tips for Setting Diet, Lifestyle, and Supplement Goals for Your Action Plan

When making your action plan, establish specific, measurable goals around diet, exercise, sleep, stress management, and supplements (if applicable). Consider:

Diet Goals:

- Reduce consumption of processed carbs, added sugars, and unhealthy fats.
- Increase intake of produce, fiber, lean protein, and healthy fats.
- Improve portion control and mindful eating habits.
- Cook more meals at home vs. eating out.

Lifestyle Goals:

- Increase moderate activity to 150+ minutes per week (e.g., brisk walking).
- Add resistance training 2-3 times per week.

- Reduce sedentary time; take movement breaks hourly.
- Achieve 7-9 hours of quality sleep nightly.
- Practice relaxation techniques to manage stress.

Supplement Goals:

- Take vitamin E, milk thistle, omega-3s, or other supplements only after discussing them with your doctor.
- Stick to the recommended dosage and timing.
- Monitor for any side effects.

Set Specifics:

- Assign numeric or actionable targets (pounds to lose, minutes of activity per week, servings of vegetables per day, etc.).
- Attach dates for when you will start and goal dates for incremental progress.
- Track metrics (weight, body fat percentage, steps, nutrition logs, sleep duration, etc.).

Revisit and revise your goals regularly. Adjust as needed based on your progress and feedback from your care team. Be realistic; small steps forward sustain motivation better than big leaps. Enlist support from loved ones. Celebrate successes along the way. Consistently working toward your diet, lifestyle, and supplement goals maximizes the reversal and prevention of fatty liver disease.

Tips on Working with Your Doctor for Ongoing Medical Care as Part of your Fatty Liver Disease Management Plan

Successfully managing fatty liver disease requires a strong partnership with your healthcare team, particularly a hepatologist or gastroenterologist. Here are some tips:

- Seek a specialist referral; a hepatologist can provide optimal evaluation and treatment guidance based on their specialized expertise with liver disease.
- Have regular follow-ups; schedule appointments every 6 to 12 months for reassessment, even if feeling well. Monitoring progress is key.
- Come prepared; beep a list of medications, supplements, symptoms, and any health changes to share at visits.
- Bring lab records; discuss trends in liver enzymes, glucose levels, lipid profile, inflammatory markers, etc. Compare to previous results.
- Ask about additional testing; inquire whether an updated ultrasound, elastography scan, MRI, or

repeat biopsy is recommended to track disease status.

- Review medications; go over any new prescriptions and OTC medications. Check for potential liver interactions.

- Discuss diet and exercise habits; be honest about adherence to recommended lifestyle changes and barriers faced. Troubleshoot shortfalls.

- Explore advanced treatments; ask about eligibility for clinical trials or medications if the disease is progressing despite lifestyle efforts.

- Provide updates; inform your provider of any hospitalizations, procedures, or other specialty care. Sign consent for coordinating care.

- Follow up on referrals; if your doctor suggests a referral to a dietitian, cardiologist, endocrinologist, or other specialist, make and keep these appointments.

Stay engaged in your care. While doctors provide guidance, you must implement the day-to-day diet, exercise, and self-care required to manage this chronic disease successfully. Ongoing medical monitoring and collaboration optimize your chances for the best possible outcome.

The Benefits of Joining a Fatty Liver Disease Support Group

In addition to working closely with your medical team, joining a fatty liver disease support group can provide immense help and encouragement on your journey. Support groups offer:

1. **Shared experiences:** Hearing from others living with the same condition provides perspective and reduces feelings of isolation. You realize you are not alone.

2. **Accountability:** Support groups promote adherence to diet, exercise, and other lifestyle changes. You want to follow through on commitments to the group.

3. **Empathy:** Fellow group members truly understand the challenges you face. Bonds form over shared struggles and victories.

4. **Insight:** Learn new perspectives on coping strategies, treatment approaches, doctor questions, etc. based on what helped others in the group.

5. **Up-to-date information:** Groups invite medical experts to present on the latest NAFLD research and clinical care standards. Stay in the know.

6. **Safe space:** Feel comfortable asking sensitive questions and expressing fears you may not want to burden loved ones with.

7. **Encouragement:** Support groups cheer you on during setbacks and celebrate successes. This motivation keeps you persistent.

8. **Hope:** Seeing others improve or even reverse their disease gives you optimism. Group progress inspires

Look for local in-person NAFLD support groups through hospitals or nonprofits. Online communities through platforms like Facebook and Reddit also allow connecting with others around the world conveniently. For children with fatty liver disease, seek out pediatric groups. Remain engaged for motivation and kinship.

Conclusion

While fatty liver disease remains a growing public health crisis, the future outlook is bright given the explosion of research underway exploring better diagnostic, preventative, and therapeutic approaches.

Advanced imaging techniques such as magnetic resonance elastography and proton density fat fraction show promise for noninvasively quantifying liver fat and fibrosis. Improved blood panels to detect biomarkers of NASH may soon reduce reliance on biopsy. Genetic testing enables risk stratification and personalized treatments.

For prevention, mass screening for NAFLD in high-risk groups could identify more cases early, when lifestyle interventions have the most significant impact. Policy and environmental changes promoting healthier eating and physical activity on a societal level could curb obesity, the key NAFLD risk factor.

Exciting pharmacological developments are emerging. Several drugs are in late-phase clinical trials for NASH-related complications, targeting pathways involved in liver inflammation, fibrosis, metabolism, and injury, with some already approved. Within a decade, effective oral agents to resolve NASH and reverse liver scarring may exist.

For advanced diseases, progress is being made with transplant options. Research shows transplanting only a portion of the liver from a deceased donor can achieve excellent outcomes when scarcity of organs is an issue. Living donor transplants are also increasingly considered for some patients.

In the interventional realm, devices that mediate liver blood flow or directly ablate liver tissue may soon provide options beyond weight-loss surgery. Investigational procedures like aspirational microbial devitalization offer hope for stabilizing late-stage disease.

While challenges remain, we now understand NAFLD's mechanisms well enough to craft targeted solutions. With continued public-private efforts and funding, the coming decade may see game-changing breakthroughs in screening, prevention, monitoring, and treatment. Fatty liver disease does not have to be our inescapable reality.

The Importance of Early Detection and Proactive Lifestyle Changes

Given the often silent progression and limited treatment options for advanced disease, early detection and proactive lifestyle changes are essential in combating the expanding fatty liver disease epidemic.

Screening high-risk individuals even without symptoms enables diagnosis at early, reversible stages rather than once cirrhosis develops. Simple blood tests and ultrasounds in those with obesity, diabetes, or metabolic syndrome can prompt further evaluation and prompt intervention. Early diagnosis provides a critical window for lifestyle changes to take effect before irreparable liver scarring occurs.

Losing just 5–10% of body weight through improved diet quality and increased physical activity can dramatically improve steatosis and stabilize NASH before fibrosis sets in. Even delaying disease progression for a few years may enable access to better future treatments. Progression to end-stage liver failure could potentially be avoided.

On a societal level, policy and environmental changes promoting healthier lifestyles for the public can curb the skyrocketing obesity rates that drive NAFLD. Limiting junk food marketing to kids, subsidizing produce, menu labeling, and building environment enhancements to encourage walking represent some initial steps.

Public awareness campaigns to educate on NAFLD risk factors and prevention are also needed. Today, few are aware that fatty liver disease is a growing epidemic and fail to recognize its risks until late complications set in. Empowering responsible self-care through accurate education is critical.

With the tidal wave of NAFLD prevalence rising each year, stemming this epidemic will require broad screening initiatives and multifaceted public health efforts. But on an individual level, we each have the power to detect this silent disease early and make impactful lifestyle choices that can alter the course of our liver health. Seize this window of opportunity before it closes.

Motivation to Kickstart Your Action Plan Against Fatty Liver Disease

Starting your fatty liver action plan now can lead to substantial health benefits.

Think of how much preventable pain and suffering you may avoid by addressing NAFLD in its early stages instead of waiting until irreversible cirrhosis develops. Take charge so you can be there as your children grow up or enjoy your retirement years to the fullest.

Picture your liver—this powerhouse organ central to many vital functions—renewed and restored by your dedication to better nutrition, more exercise, and self-care. Your whole body will reap the effects of enhanced liver health.

Remember, you can make different choices. By replacing processed foods with fresh produce, soda with water, and sedentary habits with walks or weight-lifting sessions, you pave the way for weight loss and reduced insulin resistance. Have faith in your ability to master new skills.

Keep in mind your why. Do you want to play with grandchildren someday comfortably? Travel to places on your bucket list? Pursue your passions unhindered by poor health. When temptation or inertia strikes, revisit your deepest motivations.

Focus on how much better you'll feel as the pounds come off and energy increases, thanks to an improved diet, activity, and sleep habits. Your attitude, outlook, and confidence will rise with your strengthening body.

Stay inspired by picturing yourself as a success story—someone who overcame adversity to regain vibrancy. You have the determination; now follow through with the plan. Boldly envision the destination as you take the first steps of the journey.

Remember, progress occurs one small win at a time rather than an overnight transformation. Stumble, adapt, and carry on. With consistency over months and years, seemingly minor daily choices accumulate into something powerful and life-changing.

No obstacle is insurmountable for the tenacious. Soon, wise choices will become second nature. You've got this. Bring to mind all those rooting for you whenever challenges arise along the way. Your hopes and dreams deserve your best effort, starting now.

The chance to alter your health trajectory awaits. Seize this day—this defining moment—to launch your fatty liver action plan. You hold the pen to script your success story.